JANET HIGGINSON

Put Insomnia to Bed

How I Hacked My Sleep to Beat Years of Insomnia

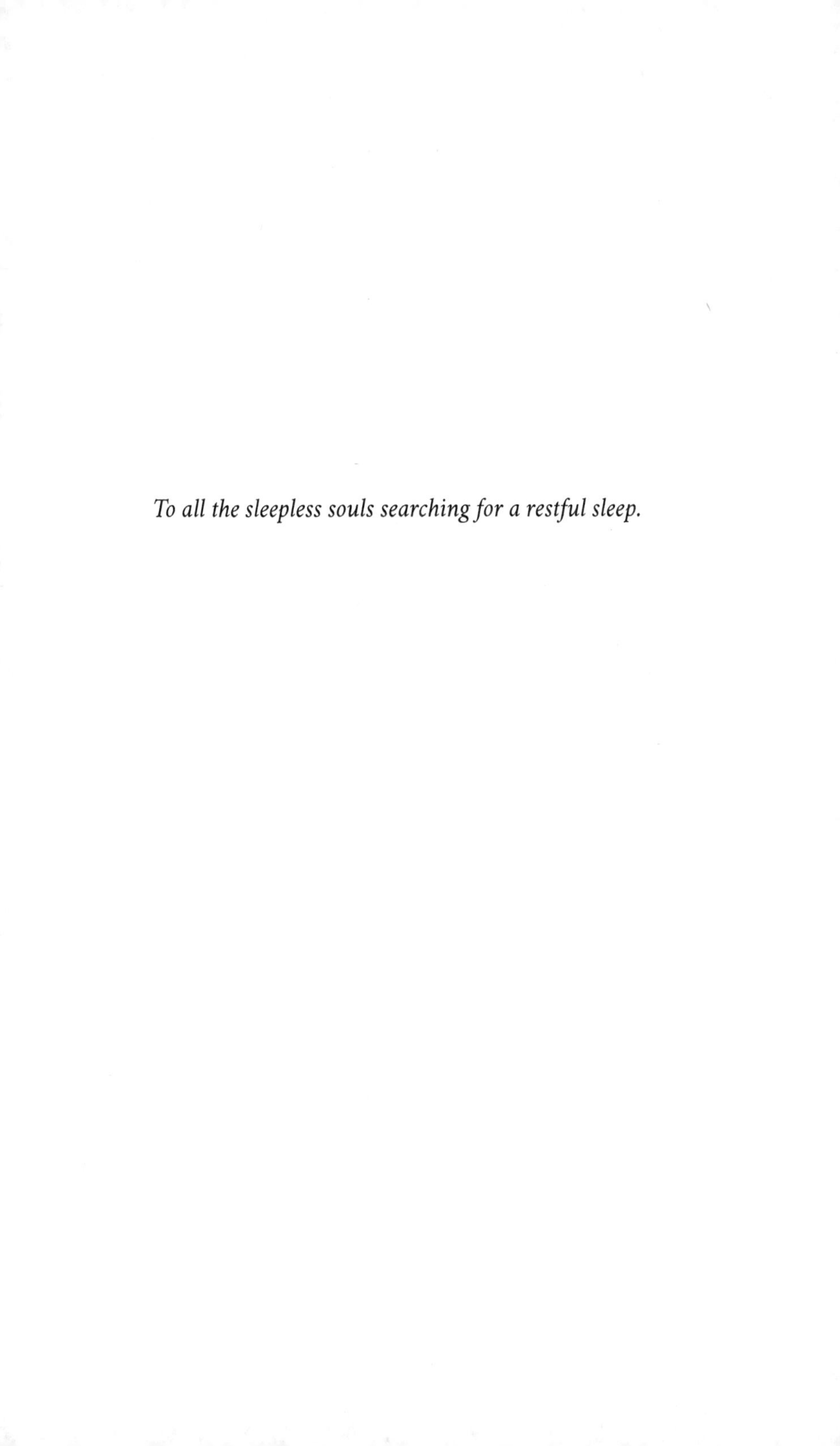

To all the sleepless souls searching for a restful sleep.

Contents

1

Introduction

Welcome to Your Journey to Restful Sleep

Imagine waking up each morning feeling refreshed, energized, and ready to take on the day. For years, that's something I couldn't imagine at all. Insomnia had its grip on me, making nights a battle and days a fog. But after countless trials and errors, I discovered the strategics that finally put my insomnia to bed. This book, "Put Insomnia to Bed: How I Hacked My Sleep to Beat Years of Insomnia" is the culmination of my journey and a guide to help you conquer sleeplessness once and for all.

Why I Wrote This Book

Sleep is a fundamental aspect of our health and well-being, yet so many of us struggle to achieve it. I know this struggle all too well. Years of tossing and turning, endless nights of staring at the ceiling, and the frustration of waking up feeling more tired than before drove me to find a solution. My own battle with insomnia inspired me to write this book. I wanted to share not only my story but also the practical, science-backed strategies that helped me regain control over my sleep. My goal is simple: to provide you with a straightforward, actionable guide to help you achieve the restful sleep you deserve.

What You'll Learn

In this book, we'll explore a variety of topics crucial to understanding and overcoming insomnia. We'll start by defining what insomnia is and how it affects your mind and body. From there, we'll delve into the impacts of artificial light and how it disrupts your natural sleep rhythms. You'll learn about the effects of caffeine and energy drinks, and why what you eat can significantly influence your sleep quality. We'll also tackle the relationship between alcohol and sleep and provide you with strategies to reset your internal clock.

Creating an optimal sleep environment is essential, and I'll guide you through building a bedroom oasis conducive to rest. We'll discuss relaxation techniques to help you unwind before bed and the importance of establishing a consistent bedtime routine. Each chapter is packed with practical advice, easy-to-follow steps, and insights that will empower you to take charge of your sleep.

How This Book Will Benefit You

By the time you finish this book, you will have a comprehensive understanding of the factors contributing to your insomnia and, more importantly, the tools to overcome it. You'll learn how to make simple yet effective changes to your daily habits, environment, and mindset that will promote better sleep. Whether you've been struggling with insomnia for years or have recently noticed your sleep quality declining, this book offers solutions tailored to your needs.

This isn't just another book filled with generic advice. It's a hands-on guide, grounded in personal experience and supported by scientific research. You'll find practical tips you can start implementing right away, and the results will speak for themselves. Restful sleep is within your reach, and this book is your roadmap to achieving it.

Now that you have a sense of what we'll be covering, it's time to dive deeper. In the next chapter, we'll explore the question: What is insomnia? We'll break down the different types of insomnia, their causes, and the impact they have on your life. Understanding the enemy is the first step in defeating it. So, let's get started on this journey to reclaim your nights and revitalize your days. Together, we'll put insomnia to bed.

2

What is Insomnia?

Understanding Insomnia: The Silent Sleep Thief

Insomnia is more than just a few sleepless nights; it's a persistent and often debilitating condition. Medically, insomnia is defined as difficulty initiating or maintaining sleep, or waking up too early and not being able to go back to sleep, occurring at least three nights per week for a minimum of three months. It can manifest as difficulty falling asleep, frequent awakenings during the night, or waking up too early in the morning. This chronic inability to achieve restorative sleep can lead to significant distress and impairment in various aspects of life.

Recognizing the Symptoms

Recognizing insomnia involves understanding its various symptoms. Common indicators include:

Difficulty Falling Asleep: Spending a prolonged amount of time trying to fall asleep at the beginning of the night.

Frequent Awakenings: Waking up multiple times during the night and having trouble getting back to sleep.

Early Morning Awakenings: Waking up too early and being unable to fall back asleep, even when still tired.

Daytime Sleepiness: Feeling excessively sleepy during the day despite spending adequate time in bed.

Cognitive Impairment: Experiencing difficulties with concentration, memory, and decision-making.

Mood Disturbances: Increased irritability, anxiety, or depression related to poor sleep.

Impacts on Daily Life

The effects of insomnia extend far beyond the night. Insufficient or poor-quality sleep can have profound impacts on daily life, including reduced productivity due to struggles with focus and task completion. Mood swings, such as increased irritability, anxiety, or depression, can strain personal and professional relationships. Chronic sleep deprivation is linked to various health problems, including weakened immune function, weight gain, hypertension, and an increased risk of cardiovascular diseases. Persistent tiredness and lack of energy can diminish the overall enjoyment of life, making everyday activities feel burdensome.

Understanding insomnia's definition, recognizing its symptoms, and acknowledging its impacts are the first steps toward addressing and managing this condition. With this knowledge, you can begin to identify whether insomnia is affecting you and take the necessary steps to improve your sleep and, consequently, your overall well-being.

In the next section, we'll explore what insomnia is not, including a look at healthy sleep cycles and how they differ from the disrupted patterns seen in insomnia.

Healthy Sleep Cycles

Understanding Healthy Sleep Cycles

Sleep is a complex and dynamic process that occurs in several stages, cycling between non-REM (NREM) and REM (rapid eye movement) sleep throughout the night. Each sleep cycle lasts about 90 to 110 minutes, and we typically go through four to six of these cycles each night.

Stages of Sleep

NREM sleep is divided into three stages:

Stage 1 (N1): This is the lightest stage of sleep, a transition period from wakefulness to sleep. It usually lasts just a few minutes. During this stage, your body starts to relax, and you can be easily awakened.

Stage 2 (N2): In this stage, your body further relaxes, with a drop in body temperature and a slowdown in heart rate and breathing. Brain activity slows, but there are brief bursts of electrical activity called sleep spindles, which are believed to play a role in consolidating memories.

Stage 3 (N3): This is deep sleep, also known as slow-wave sleep. It's the most restorative stage, essential for physical recovery and growth, bolstering the immune system, and repairing tissues. This stage is crucial for feeling refreshed in the morning.

REM sleep, the final stage in the cycle, is where most dreaming occurs. It plays a key role in cognitive functions such as memory, learning, and creativity. During REM sleep, brain activity increases, nearing levels seen when you are awake, but your muscles remain relaxed to prevent acting out dreams.

Quantity and Quality of Sleep

Healthy adults typically need seven to nine hours of sleep per night. The quality of sleep is equally important; uninterrupted cycles of NREM and REM sleep ensure the body and brain get the rest needed to function optimally. Disruptions in these cycles can lead to impaired cognitive function, weakened immune response, and overall reduced health and well-being.

The Impact of Healthy Sleep

Achieving and maintaining a healthy sleep cycle has profound effects on daily life. It enhances cognitive functions, such as memory and decision-making, supports emotional regulation, and fosters physical health by aiding muscle repair, tissue growth, and immune function. Consistent, high-quality sleep can improve mood, increase productivity, and enhance the overall quality of life.

Understanding the stages of sleep and their functions helps underscore the importance of both sleep quantity and quality.

When to See Your Doctor

While this book offers practical strategies for overcoming insomnia, there are instances when professional medical advice is necessary. If you experience persistent sleep issues that significantly impact your daily life or suspect an underlying health condition, it's crucial to consult a doctor. Here are some specific conditions that warrant medical attention:

Sleep Apnea

Sleep apnea is a serious sleep disorder characterized by repeated interruptions in breathing during sleep. These interruptions can last from a few seconds to minutes and may occur multiple times per hour. Common symptoms include loud snoring, gasping for air during sleep, and waking up with a dry mouth or headache. If you suspect you have sleep apnea, it's essential to seek medical evaluation, as untreated sleep apnea can lead to severe health issues, including heart disease, high blood pressure, and stroke.

Stress and Anxiety

Chronic stress and anxiety are common sleep disruptors. When your mind is preoccupied with worries or racing thoughts, falling and staying asleep can become challenging. Persistent stress can lead to insomnia, creating a cycle where lack of sleep exacerbates stress levels. If you find that stress or anxiety significantly interferes with your sleep despite trying various relaxation techniques, it may be beneficial to speak with a healthcare professional. They can help identify the underlying causes and recommend appropriate treatments, which may include therapy or medication.

Depression

Depression often goes hand-in-hand with sleep disturbances. People with depression may experience difficulty falling asleep, staying asleep, or waking up too early. Conversely, excessive sleepiness and prolonged sleep duration can also be symptoms of depression. If you notice changes in your sleep patterns accompanied by feelings of sadness, hopelessness, or a loss of interest in daily activities, it's important to seek medical advice. Effective treatment for depression can improve both your mental health and sleep quality.

Menopause

For women, menopause and the transition leading up to it (perimenopause) can cause significant sleep disturbances. Hormonal fluctuations, particularly decreases in estrogen and progesterone, can lead to night sweats, hot flashes, and mood swings, all of which can disrupt sleep. If menopausal symptoms are affecting your sleep, consult with your doctor. They can discuss potential treatments, such as hormone replacement therapy (HRT) or other medications and lifestyle adjustments, to help manage symptoms and improve sleep quality.

Other Health Conditions

Other medical conditions, such as chronic pain, gastrointestinal disorders, and neurological conditions, can also impact sleep. For instance, restless legs syndrome (RLS) and periodic limb movement disorder (PLMD) cause uncomfortable sensations in the legs and involuntary leg movements during sleep, leading to frequent awakenings. If you have any chronic health issues that you suspect are interfering with your sleep, it's important to address these with your healthcare provider. They can help manage these conditions more effectively, potentially improving your sleep in the process.

When Self-Help Isn't Enough

If you've tried the strategies in this book and still struggle with sleep, or if your sleep problems are severe, don't hesitate to seek medical help. Persistent insomnia can be a sign of a more serious underlying issue, and professional guidance can provide the support you need to identify and treat these problems effectively. Remember, prioritizing your sleep is a crucial step toward overall health and well-being.

In the next chapter, we'll explore how artificial light impacts your sleep and what you can do to mitigate its effects. Understanding and addressing external factors that influence sleep is key to creating an environment conducive to rest. Let's continue this journey to better sleep together.

3

How Artificial Light Messes With Your Sleep

Light After Sunset and Melatonin Production

Impact of Light Exposure on Humans

Light exposure plays a crucial role in regulating the body's internal clock, known as the circadian rhythm. This rhythm influences the sleep-wake cycle, hormone release, eating habits, and other bodily functions. When light enters the eyes, it signals the brain's suprachiasmatic nucleus (SCN), which then adjusts the production of melatonin, the hormone responsible for making us feel sleepy. During the day, light exposure keeps melatonin levels low, promoting alertness and wakefulness. However, as evening approaches and natural light decreases, the SCN signals the pineal gland to increase melatonin production, preparing the body for sleep.

Detrimental Effects of Light Exposure After Sunset

Exposure to artificial light after sunset can disrupt this natural process, leading to difficulties in falling and staying asleep. Artificial light, especially blue light from screens and LED lights, mimics daylight and confuses the brain into thinking it is still daytime. This misalignment can significantly reduce melatonin production in the evening, delaying sleep onset and disrupting the overall quality of sleep.

The impact of light on sleep is well-documented. According to the Sleep Foundation, even low levels of artificial light can suppress melatonin production. This suppression can lead to an increase in alertness and a delay in the body's readiness for sleep. Over time, this disruption can result in chronic sleep problems and contribute to long-term health issues, such as increased risk for cardiovascular diseases, obesity, and mental health disorders.

Natural light exposure during the day and darkness at night are vital for maintaining a healthy circadian rhythm. When artificial light extends daylight into the evening, it can cause several issues:

Delayed Sleep Phase: Prolonged light exposure in the evening can shift the sleep phase later, making it harder to fall asleep at a desired time. This can lead to insufficient sleep duration, especially if wake-up times cannot be adjusted accordingly.

Reduced Sleep Quality: Lower melatonin levels at night can affect the depth and quality of sleep. People might experience lighter sleep stages and reduced amounts of restorative deep and REM sleep, leading to less refreshing sleep.

Increased Alertness: Blue light, in particular, is known to increase alertness. This heightened state of wakefulness can make it more challenging to unwind and relax before bedtime.

Creating an environment that mimics natural light patterns—bright during the day and dim or dark in the evening—can help align the body's internal clock with the natural day-night cycle, promoting better sleep and overall health.

In the next section, we will explore the specific impact of blue light from technology and strategies to mitigate its effects on sleep.

Blue Light from Technology

The impact of blue light on sleep cannot be overstated, particularly in our technology-driven world. Blue light, a high-energy visible light with a short wavelength, is emitted in significant amounts by various technological devices such as TVs, LED lights, computers, and cell phones. This type of light has been found to have a profound impact on sleep patterns and overall sleep quality.

Blue light exposure, especially in the evening, can severely disrupt the body's natural circadian rhythm. This disruption occurs because blue light mimics the effects of daylight, signaling the brain to stay awake and alert. The primary way blue light affects sleep is by inhibiting the production of melatonin, the hormone that regulates sleep. Reduced melatonin levels can delay sleep onset, shorten total sleep duration, and decrease the quality of sleep by interfering with deep and REM sleep stages.

Modern televisions and LED light bulbs emit large amounts of blue light, and watching TV late into the night can keep your brain stimulated and delay the onset of sleep. The screens of computers, tablets, and smartphones are also significant sources of blue light. The close proximity of these devices to the eyes further intensifies their impact on melatonin suppression and circadian rhythm disruption.

Apart from the physiological effects of blue light, the content consumed on these devices plays a critical role in sleep disruption. Social media platforms and games are designed to be engaging and can be highly addictive. The constant notifications, the urge to check updates, and the immersive nature of games can significantly extend screen time, reducing the time available for sleep. The interactive and rewarding aspects of these platforms can make it challenging to disconnect and wind down before bedtime, further exacerbating sleep problems.

Understanding the impact of blue light and the addictive nature of modern technology is essential for improving sleep quality. To mitigate these effects, consider using blue light blocking technology. Many devices now come with night mode or blue light filter settings that reduce the amount of blue light emitted. Blue light blocking glasses are also available and can be worn in the evening. Limiting screen time before bed, ideally avoiding screens at least one hour before bedtime, allows your body to start producing melatonin naturally. Engaging in relaxing activities such as reading a book (preferably a physical one) or practicing mindfulness can also help. Creating a tech-free bedroom by keeping electronic devices out of the room can further promote a sleep-conducive environment and reduce both blue light exposure and the temptation to check social media or play games late into the night.

By being mindful of blue light exposure and the content consumed on electronic devices, you can take significant steps toward improving your sleep quality and overall health.

Using Red Light and Blue Light Blockers to Improve Sleep

The Role of Red Light

Red light has emerged as a beneficial option for evening lighting, primarily because it has minimal impact on melatonin production. Unlike blue light, which mimics daylight and can suppress melatonin, red light does not interfere with the body's natural sleep signals. Research suggests that red light exposure in the evening can help maintain the circadian rhythm and promote better sleep. Anecdotal evidence from individuals who have switched to red light bulbs or lamps in their bedrooms indicates improvements in falling asleep faster and experiencing more restful sleep. This is because red light creates a calm and relaxing environment, which is conducive to winding down and preparing the body for sleep.

Benefits of Blue Light Blocking Glasses

Blue light blocking glasses are designed to filter out blue wavelengths of light, reducing their impact on melatonin production. These glasses can be particularly useful in the evening when exposure to screens and artificial lighting is hard to avoid. By wearing blue light blocking glasses, individuals can continue their evening activities, such as reading on a tablet or watching TV, without significantly disrupting their sleep patterns. Studies have shown that using blue light blocking glasses can improve sleep quality and duration, especially in people who are sensitive to light or have sleep disorders. Not all blue light blocking glasses are the same, so make sure you invest in a quality pair that blocks the most blue light.

Anecdotal Evidence and Personal Experiences

Many individuals who have incorporated red light and blue light blockers into their nightly routines report noticeable improvements in their sleep. For instance, people who switch to red light bulbs in their bedside lamps often find it easier to fall asleep and stay asleep throughout the night. Similarly, those who wear blue light blocking glasses for a couple of hours before bedtime often experience fewer difficulties with sleep onset and enjoy more consistent, high-quality sleep. These personal accounts, combined with scientific research, underscore the effectiveness of these interventions in promoting better sleep health.

Implementing Red Light and Blue Light Blockers

To make the most of these strategies, consider the following tips:

Use Red Light Bulbs: Replace standard light bulbs in your bedroom and other areas where you spend your evenings with red light bulbs. This creates a soothing atmosphere that supports melatonin production and helps signal to your body that it's time to prepare for sleep

Wear Blue Light Blocking Glasses: Start wearing blue light blocking glasses about two hours before your intended bedtime. This can significantly reduce the blue light exposure from screens and artificial lighting, allowing your body to produce melatonin naturally.

Combine Strategies: For optimal results, combine the use of red light and blue light blockers. Create an evening routine that minimizes exposure to blue light while incorporating red light to maintain a relaxing environment.

By understanding and utilizing the benefits of red light and blue light blocking technology, you can significantly enhance your sleep quality.

Total Darkness for Sleeping

Creating an environment of total darkness is one of the most effective ways to enhance sleep quality. Darkness signals to the body that it is time to rest, promoting the production of melatonin, the hormone responsible for regulating sleep. Here are several strategies to achieve a completely dark sleeping environment.

Using Blackout Curtains or Window Coverings

Blackout curtains or window coverings are essential for blocking out external light sources, such as streetlights, car headlights, or early morning sunlight. These curtains are made from heavy, opaque materials that prevent light from entering the room, creating a dark and conducive environment for sleep. Installing these curtains can help maintain a consistent sleep-wake cycle, allowing you to fall asleep more easily and stay asleep longer.

Blocking All Sources of Light

Even small amounts of light from electronic devices can disrupt sleep by interfering with melatonin production. Alarm clocks with bright displays, LED indicators on smoke detectors, and light from outlets or chargers can all contribute to light pollution in the bedroom. To address this, consider using blackout covers for alarm clocks or choosing models with dimmable displays. For other devices, use electrical tape or specially designed light-blocking stickers to cover any LED indicators. These small adjustments can significantly reduce unwanted light and create a darker, more restful sleep environment.

Keeping TV and Cell Phone Out of the Bedroom

Removing TVs and cell phones from the bedroom is another crucial step in achieving total darkness. The screens of these devices emit blue light, which can inhibit melatonin production and delay sleep onset. Additionally, the temptation to use these devices before bed can prolong exposure to light and stimulate the brain, making it harder to wind down. If you use your cell phone as an alarm clock, consider placing it in a nearby room where you can still hear it but are not exposed to its light. Later in this book, we will discuss strategies to limit light exposure from your cell phone during sleep, ensuring that you can maintain a dark environment while still using it for essential functions like alarms.

Additional Tips for a Darker Sleep Environment

Seal Light Leaks: Ensure that no light seeps in around the edges of blackout curtains or through cracks in the door. Using draft stoppers or weather stripping can help seal these gaps.

Adjust Nightlights: If nightlights are necessary for safety, choose those with red bulbs, as red light has the least impact on melatonin production and sleep cycles.

Consider Sleep Masks: For individuals who cannot fully darken their rooms, sleep masks can provide an additional layer of darkness by covering the eyes and blocking out remaining light sources.

By striving for a completely dark sleep environment, you can significantly enhance the quality of your sleep. These adjustments help maintain melatonin levels, support a healthy circadian rhythm, and create a tranquil space conducive to restful sleep.

Room Temperature

The Impact of Room Temperature on Sleep

Room temperature plays a critical role in the quality of your sleep. The human body has a natural temperature cycle that aligns with the sleep-wake rhythm, typically dropping in temperature as it prepares for sleep and reaching its lowest point in the early morning hours. This decline in core body temperature is crucial for initiating and maintaining sleep. When the room temperature is too high or too low, it can interfere with this natural process, making it harder to fall asleep and stay asleep throughout the night.

Sleeping in a room that is too warm can lead to restlessness, frequent awakenings, and reduced time spent in the deep and REM stages of sleep, which are essential for physical and mental restoration. Conversely, while cooler temperatures generally promote sleep, a room that is excessively cold can cause discomfort and disrupt sleep as your body struggles to maintain a comfortable core temperature.

Optimal Room Temperature for Sleep

Research suggests that the optimal room temperature for sleep is between 60 and 67 degrees Fahrenheit (15 to 19 degrees Celsius). This range supports the natural drop in body temperature that facilitates sleep onset and maintenance. A cooler environment helps reduce the body's core temperature more effectively, signaling to the brain that it is time to sleep. Additionally, cooler temperatures can prevent overheating and sweating, which can lead to discomfort and sleep disturbances.

Tips for Achieving the Optimal Sleep Temperature

To achieve and maintain the optimal room temperature for sleep, consider the following tips:

Use a Thermostat: Adjust your thermostat to maintain a consistent temperature within the optimal range. Programmable thermostats can be set to lower the temperature automatically in the evening and raise it in the morning. If you don't have a separate thermostat in your bedroom consider placing a cheap wall mounted thermometer near your bed. You might find the temperature set on your living room thermostat is off by several degrees from the bedroom.

Bedding Choices: Choose bedding and sleepwear that help regulate your body temperature. Lightweight, breathable fabrics such as cotton or linen are ideal for promoting airflow and preventing overheating.

Fans and Air Conditioning: Use fans or air conditioning to keep the air circulating and maintain a cool environment.

Layering: Use layers of bedding that can be added or removed as needed to adjust to temperature changes during the night. This flexibility allows you to maintain comfort without overheating.

Ventilation: Ensure proper ventilation in your bedroom by opening windows or using a ventilation system to allow fresh air to circulate, helping to regulate temperature naturally.

By optimizing your room temperature, you can create a sleep environment that enhances the natural processes of your body, leading to better sleep quality and overall hcalth.

4

Caffeine and Energy Drinks

Caffeine and Its Impact on Sleep

Caffeine is a central nervous system stimulant widely consumed around the world, primarily in coffee, tea, soft drinks, and various medications. It works by blocking the effects of adenosine, a brain chemical involved in promoting sleep, thereby increasing alertness and reducing the feeling of fatigue. While this can be beneficial during the day, caffeine consumption, especially in the hours leading up to bedtime, can significantly disrupt sleep.

Effects of Caffeine Based on Consumption, Amount and Timing

The impact of caffeine on sleep largely depends on how much is consumed and when it is consumed. Consuming high amounts of caffeine can lead to a more pronounced disruption in sleep. Studies have shown that even a moderate intake of caffeine (200 mg, roughly equivalent to a cup of coffee) can reduce sleep efficiency and total sleep time, especially if consumed later in the day. The Sleep Foundation points out that caffeine can remain in the bloodstream for several hours, with a half life of about five to six hours. This means that caffeine consumed in the late afternoon or evening can still be active in the system at bedtime, making it difficult to fall asleep and stay asleep.

For example, drinking a cup of coffee at 4 PM might still have a quarter of its caffeine content in your system by 10 PM. This lingering caffeine can interfere with the natural decline in alertness that facilitates sleep onset. Additionally, research from PubMed indicates that caffeine can reduce the amount of slow-wave sleep (deep sleep) you get, which is essential for physical and mental restoration. People who consume large amounts of caffeine, or who are particularly sensitive to its effects, might find themselves tossing and turning, unable to achieve a restful night's sleep.

Guidelines for Caffeine Consumption

To minimize the negative impact of caffeine on sleep, it is advisable to limit caffeine intake, especially in the afternoon and evening. Aim to consume caffeine primarily in the morning and early afternoon, allowing sufficient time for your body to metabolize it before bedtime. If you are particularly sensitive to caffeine, consider reducing your overall intake or switching to decaffeinated beverages.

While caffeine can be a helpful stimulant during the day, its consumption should be carefully managed to avoid disrupting sleep. By understanding the timing and amount of caffeine intake, individuals can better align their consumption habits with their sleep needs, ensuring they get the restorative rest necessary for overall health and well-being.

Energy Drinks for the Win?

Impact of Energy Drinks on the Body and Sleep

Energy drinks are popular for their ability to provide a quick boost of energy and alertness. These beverages typically contain high levels of caffeine along with other stimulants like guarana, taurine, and ginseng. While they might offer a temporary energy boost, their impact on the body and sleep can be quite detrimental.

Energy drinks often contain caffeine levels far exceeding those found in coffee or tea. For example, a single can of some energy drinks can contain up to 500 mg of caffeine, equivalent to about five cups of coffee. This high caffeine content can lead to increased heart rate and blood pressure, making it difficult for the body to relax and prepare for sleep. The stimulants in energy drinks not only delay sleep onset but also reduce the total sleep time and sleep efficiency. According to research cited by Health.com, individuals who consume more energy drinks report poorer sleep quality and increased levels of daytime sleepiness compared to those who consume fewer or no energy drinks.

Why Energy Drinks Are Generally Bad for You

Beyond their impact on sleep, energy drinks pose several health risks. The combination of high caffeine content and other stimulants can lead to various cardiovascular issues, including palpitations, arrhythmias, and in severe cases, heart attacks. The sugar content in many energy drinks can also contribute to weight gain, insulin resistance, and dental problems. Additionally, the excessive consumption of these beverages has been linked to increased anxiety, agitation, and even potential dependency.

Energy drinks can create a vicious cycle of dependency, where poor sleep quality leads to increased consumption of these beverages to combat daytime fatigue. This, in turn, further disrupts sleep, perpetuating the cycle. The high levels of caffeine and sugar provide a short-term energy spike followed by a crash, which can exacerbate feelings of tiredness and prompt further consumption of energy drinks.

Guidelines for Reducing Energy Drink Consumption

To improve sleep quality and overall health, it is advisable to limit the consumption of energy drinks. Instead, opt for healthier alternatives like water, herbal teas, or natural juices. If a caffeine boost is needed, moderate coffee or tea consumption earlier in the day is a better option. Maintaining a balanced diet, regular exercise, and good sleep hygiene practices can naturally enhance energy levels without the need for stimulants.

Though energy drinks might seem like a convenient solution for combating fatigue, their impact on sleep and overall health is largely negative. Understanding these effects can help individuals make more informed choices about their consumption habits, leading to better sleep quality and improved well-being. In the next chapter, we will explore how diet influences sleep and provide strategies for eating in a way that supports restful sleep.

5

You Sleep What You Eat

Timing is Everything

Optimal Timing for Eating and Sleep

The timing of your meals can significantly affect your sleep quality. For optimal sleep, it's best to finish eating at least two to three hours before bedtime. This allows your body enough time to digest the food before you go to sleep, reducing the risk of discomfort and indigestion that can keep you awake. Eating your largest meal earlier in the day, such as at breakfast or lunch, can also help regulate your metabolism and support a healthy circadian rhythm.

Eating a heavy meal right before bed can cause your body to work on digestion instead of preparing for sleep. This can lead to issues such as acid reflux or heartburn, especially if you lie down too soon after eating. Lighter meals in the evening are recommended to minimize these risks. Foods rich in complex carbohydrates, lean proteins, and healthy fats can promote a more restful sleep, while heavy, spicy, or fatty foods can be more disruptive.

Worst Times to Eat for Sleep

Consuming meals or snacks late at night can interfere with your ability to fall asleep and stay asleep. Eating close to bedtime can keep your body in an active state, digesting food when it should be winding down for rest. This can result in fragmented sleep and a feeling of tiredness upon waking. Additionally, late-night eating can disrupt your circadian rhythm, leading to misalignment between your sleep-wake cycle and your eating habits.

Studies show that late-night eating is associated with poorer sleep quality and can contribute to conditions such as insomnia. It's also linked to an increased risk of metabolic disorders, as the body's ability to process glucose decreases at night. To avoid these issues, try to make a light dinner your last meal of the day and avoid heavy or sugary snacks before bed.

By understanding the best and worst times to eat in relation to sleep, you can adjust your eating schedule to promote better sleep quality. Aim to have your last meal a few hours before bedtime and focus on lighter, more easily digestible foods in the evening.

Food Additives and Food Sensitivities

The Impact of Food Additives on Sleep

Food additives are substances added to foods to enhance flavor, appearance, or shelf life. While these additives can make foods more convenient and appealing, they can also have negative effects on sleep.

Common additives such as monosodium glutamate (MSG), artificial colors, and preservatives have been linked to various health issues, including sleep disturbances.

MSG, often found in processed foods and Chinese cuisine, can cause reactions in sensitive individuals, including headaches, palpitations, and feelings of restlessness, which can interfere with sleep. Similarly, artificial food colorings, especially those derived from petroleum like Red 40 and Yellow 5, have been associated with hyperactivity and sleep problems in both children and adults. Preservatives like sodium benzoate and nitrates, commonly found in processed meats and packaged foods, can also contribute to sleep disruptions by causing indigestion, increased heart rate, and other adverse reactions.

Unknown Food Sensitivities and Sleep

Food sensitivities or intolerances can significantly impact sleep quality, often in ways that people may not immediately recognize. Unlike food allergies, which provoke an immediate and often severe reaction, food sensitivities can cause delayed and subtler symptoms such as digestive issues, headaches, and fatigue. These symptoms can disrupt sleep by causing discomfort and restlessness during the night.

For instance, lactose intolerance can lead to bloating, gas, and diarrhea, especially when dairy products are consumed close to bedtime. Gluten sensitivity, common in individuals with celiac disease or non-celiac gluten sensitivity, can cause gastrointestinal discomfort and inflammatory responses that disturb sleep. Other common culprits include caffeine, which can be hidden in some foods and beverages, and high-histamine foods, which can exacerbate conditions like acid reflux or histamine intolerance, leading to sleep disturbances.

Identifying and Managing Food Additives and Sensitivities

To identify food additives and sensitivities that might be affecting your sleep, it can be helpful to keep a food diary. Note what you eat and drink, along with any symptoms you experience, particularly those related to sleep. This can help you pinpoint specific foods or additives that trigger adverse reactions.

Eliminating or reducing intake of processed foods and opting for whole, natural foods can minimize exposure to potentially harmful additives. If you suspect a food sensitivity, consider an elimination diet, where you remove suspected foods from your diet for a period and then gradually reintroduce them to observe any reactions. Consulting with a healthcare professional, such as a dietitian or allergist, can also provide guidance and testing to identify and manage food sensitivities effectively.

In summary, both food additives and unknown food sensitivities can disrupt sleep, leading to a range of sleep-related issues. By being mindful of what you consume and identifying any problematic foods, you can take steps to improve your sleep quality. For further information on food additives and sensitivities, refer to continuously updated resources provided by health organizations and nutrition experts.

Hydration

The Importance of Proper Hydration for Restful Sleep

Hydration plays a crucial role in maintaining overall health and well-being, including the quality of your sleep. Proper hydration helps regulate body temperature, maintain metabolic processes, and support cognitive functions. Dehydration, on the other hand, can lead to discomfort, such as dry mouth and nasal passages, muscle cramps, and headaches, all of which can disrupt sleep and prevent you from getting a restful night's rest.

According to the Sleep Foundation, maintaining adequate hydration levels during the day can support better sleep by ensuring that your body functions optimally. Adequate hydration supports the body's natural processes and can prevent the physical discomforts that often lead to restless nights.

Tapering Off Hydration Before Bedtime

While staying hydrated throughout the day is essential, it is equally important to manage fluid intake as bedtime approaches. Drinking too much water or other fluids in the evening can lead to frequent trips to the bathroom during the night, disrupting sleep continuity and quality. Nocturia, or nighttime urination, is a common issue that can fragment sleep and make it challenging to enter the deeper stages of sleep necessary for physical and mental restoration.

To minimize the risk of nocturia, it is advisable to start tapering off fluid intake about two to three hours before bedtime. This allows your body time to process and excrete excess fluids before you go to sleep. Additionally, consider reducing the intake of diuretic beverages, such as caffeinated drinks and alcohol, in the evening as, among other things, these can increase urine production and contribute to nighttime awakenings.

Practical Tips for Managing Hydration

To maintain optimal hydration without compromising sleep quality, follow these practical tips:

Hydrate Early in the Day: Focus on drinking the majority of your fluids earlier in the day. Aim to meet most of your hydration needs by mid-afternoon to reduce the need for large fluid intake in the evening.

Monitor Fluid Intake: Keep track of your fluid consumption, especially in the hours leading up to bedtime. If you find yourself waking up frequently at night to urinate, consider adjusting your evening hydration habits.

Choose Hydrating Foods: Incorporate water-rich foods into your diet, such as fruits and vegetables, which can help maintain hydration levels without requiring excessive fluid intake.

Balance Electrolytes: Ensure that your hydration strategy includes electrolyte balance, particularly if you engage in activities that cause heavy sweating. Electrolytes such as sodium, potassium, and magnesium help the body retain fluids and maintain hydration without overloading the bladder.

Create a Routine: Establish a consistent hydration routine that works for your lifestyle and sleep schedule. By making conscious choices about when and how much to drink, you can support both hydration and sleep quality.

Proper hydration is vital for overall health and can significantly impact sleep quality. By managing your fluid intake wisely, especially as bedtime approaches, you can minimize sleep disruptions and promote a more restful night's sleep. In the next section, we will explore the effects of stimulants in food on sleep and how to manage their consumption for better sleep hygiene.

For more detailed information on hydration and sleep, refer to resources provided by the Sleep Foundation and other reputable health organizations.

6

Alcohol and Sleep Quality

The Impacts of Alcohol on Sleep

Alcohol is often consumed to help unwind and induce sleepiness, but its effects on sleep quality are mostly negative. While alcohol can help you fall asleep more quickly due to its sedative properties, it disrupts the sleep cycle and reduces overall sleep quality.

Disruption of Sleep Stages

Alcohol affects the architecture of sleep by altering the balance of sleep stages. Typically, sleep progresses through three stages of non-rapid eye movement (NREM) sleep and one stage of rapid eye movement (REM) sleep, cycling through these stages every 90 to 120 minutes. Alcohol consumption increases the proportion of deep sleep (NREM stage 3) during the first half of the night, which might seem beneficial at first. However, as the body metabolizes the alcohol, sleep becomes lighter and more fragmented in the second half of the night. This shift leads to a reduction in REM sleep, which is crucial for cognitive functions like memory consolidation and emotional regulation.

As alcohol wears off, the sedative effects diminish, leading to increased wakefulness and sleep fragmentation. This disruption often results in frequent awakenings and a feeling of unrefreshed sleep the next day. The fragmented sleep pattern caused by alcohol can reduce the restorative quality of sleep, leaving you feeling groggy and tired despite spending enough time in bed

Long-Term Effects and Sleep Disorders

Chronic use of alcohol can exacerbate sleep disorders such as insomnia and obstructive sleep apnea (OSA). Alcohol relaxes the muscles in the throat, increasing the likelihood of airway obstruction in individuals with OSA. It can also worsen snoring and other breathing-related sleep issues. Over time, heavy alcohol use can lead to a vicious cycle where poor sleep quality prompts further alcohol use as a sleep aid, perpetuating sleep disturbances and potentially leading to dependence.

Guidelines for Alcohol Consumption

To minimize the negative impact of alcohol on sleep, it is recommended to avoid consuming alcohol at least three hours before bedtime. This allows your body to metabolize the alcohol, reducing its disruptive effects on the sleep cycle. For better sleep hygiene, consider limiting alcohol intake and exploring alternative relaxation methods such as herbal teas, meditation, and establishing a consistent bedtime routine.

Understanding the impacts of alcohol on sleep can help you make informed decisions about your drinking habits, leading to improved sleep quality and overall well-being.

7

Resetting Your Internal Clock

Our Circadian Rhythms Are Out of Whack

Circadian rhythms are the natural, internal processes that regulate the sleep-wake cycle and repeat roughly every 24 hours. These rhythms are influenced by external cues like light and temperature. However, modern lifestyle factors such as artificial light, technology, and shift work have significantly disrupted these natural cycles.

Artificial Light

Artificial light is one of the primary disruptors of our circadian rhythms. Before the advent of electric lighting, people's sleep patterns were closely aligned with the natural light-dark cycle of the day. However, with the widespread use of artificial light, especially after sunset, our exposure to light has extended well beyond the natural daylight hours. This prolonged light exposure can interfere with the production of melatonin, the hormone that signals to our bodies that it is time to sleep.

The blue light emitted by LED and fluorescent lights is particularly problematic, as it is more effective at suppressing melatonin production compared to other wavelengths of light.

Technology

The pervasive use of technology further compounds the problem. Devices such as smartphones, tablets, computers, and televisions emit blue light, which can significantly disrupt our circadian rhythms. The light from these screens can delay the onset of sleep by reducing melatonin production, making it harder to fall asleep at the desired time. Additionally, engaging with stimulating content on these devices, such as social media, games, or work-related activities, can keep the brain active and alert, further hindering the natural winding-down process that precedes sleep.

Shift Work

Shift work presents another significant challenge to maintaining healthy circadian rhythms. Many jobs require individuals to work during the night and sleep during the day, which is contrary to the body's natural inclination to be awake during daylight and asleep after sunset. This misalignment can lead to chronic sleep disorders, decreased sleep quality, and a range of health issues including increased risk of cardiovascular diseases, obesity, and mental health disorders. Shift workers often experience difficulties in maintaining a consistent sleep schedule, which exacerbates the disruption of their circadian rhythms.

These modern lifestyle factors collectively contribute to the misalignment of our natural circadian rhythms, leading to difficulties in falling asleep, staying asleep, and waking up feeling rested. Understanding these disruptions is the first step towards implementing strategies to reset and maintain a healthy sleep-wake cycle. In the following sections, we will explore practical solutions to mitigate these disruptions and promote better sleep health.

Stimulant Cycle

Modern lifestyles often create a cycle of using stimulants like caffeine and energy drinks to wake up and stay alert during the day, followed by relying on sleep aids to fall asleep at night. This cycle can significantly disrupt natural sleep patterns and overall health.

The Cycle of Stimulants and Sleep Aids

Many people start their day with a boost from caffeine, found in coffee, tea, and energy drinks. Caffeine works by blocking adenosine receptors in the brain, which helps reduce the feeling of fatigue and increases alertness. However, consuming too much caffeine, especially later in the day, can interfere with the ability to fall asleep at night. The half-life of caffeine is about five to six hours, meaning it can remain in your system long after consumption, affecting your sleep quality.

To counteract the stimulating effects of caffeine and combat the resulting sleep difficulties, some individuals turn to sleep aids, including over-the-counter medications, prescription drugs, and supplements like melatonin. While these aids can help induce sleep in the short term, they can become problematic if used regularly. Dependence on sleep aids can develop, leading to tolerance and reduced effectiveness over time. Additionally, using sleep aids without addressing underlying sleep hygiene issues can perpetuate the cycle of poor sleep quality and reliance on stimulants.

Sleep Aids and Melatonin

While sleep aids, including melatonin supplements, can be useful for occasional sleep disturbances, regular use can be problematic. Melatonin is a hormone naturally produced by the body to regulate the sleep-wake cycle. Supplementing with melatonin can help in cases of jet lag or temporary sleep disruptions, but overuse can lead to dependence and disrupt the body's natural melatonin production. Other sleep aids, such as prescription medications, can carry risks of side effects, tolerance, and dependence. It is important to use these aids sparingly and under the guidance of a healthcare professional.

Breaking the stimulant cycle involves adopting healthier sleep habits and reducing reliance on substances to regulate wakefulness and sleep. By cutting out energy drinks, limiting caffeine intake, and using sleep aids judiciously, you can support a more natural and restorative sleep pattern.

Natural Light Reset

Resetting your internal clock through exposure to natural light is an effective way to synchronize your circadian rhythms with the natural day-night cycle. This process involves a daily protocol of watching the sunrise and sunset, preferably outside. Here's how you can implement this natural light reset protocol to improve your sleep patterns and overall well-being.

Morning Light Exposure

Watch the Sunrise: Begin your day by watching the sunrise. Exposure to natural light in the morning helps signal to your brain that it is time to wake up and be alert. This early morning light is rich in blue wavelengths, which are particularly effective at suppressing melatonin production and shifting your circadian rhythm to match the natural light-dark cycle.

Spend Time Outdoors: After watching the sunrise, try to spend at least 30 minutes outside. Engage in activities such as walking, jogging, or simply sitting in natural light. Morning light exposure not only helps reset your internal clock but also boosts mood and energy levels due to increased serotonin production.

Evening Light Exposure

Watch the Sunset: As the day winds down, make it a habit to watch the sunset. The warm, amber light of the setting sun signals to your brain that it is time to start winding down and preparing for sleep. This natural light exposure in the evening helps reinforce the natural decrease in light exposure as the day progresses, promoting the production of melatonin.

Reduce Artificial Light Exposure: After sunset, minimize exposure to artificial light, especially blue light from screens and electronic devices. Use dim, warm lighting in your home and consider using blue light blocking glasses if you need to use electronic devices. This helps maintain the natural progression towards darkness, encouraging your body to produce melatonin and prepare for sleep.

Daily Protocol

Morning: Spend at least 30 minutes outside in natural light, ideally watching the sunrise or being exposed to early morning sunlight.

Evening: Watch the sunset and reduce exposure to artificial light afterward. Aim to spend time outdoors during the evening light to signal to your body that it is time to wind down.

Consistency: Consistency is key! Make this natural light exposure a daily routine to effectively reset your internal clock. Regular exposure to natural light at consistent times helps reinforce your body's circadian rhythm, making it easier to fall asleep and wake up at the desired times.

By following this natural light reset protocol, you can help realign your circadian rhythms with the natural day-night cycle, leading to improved sleep quality and overall health.

8

Relaxation Strategies

Relaxation strategies play a crucial role in calming the mind and regulating the nervous system to prepare for sleep. This chapter outlines various techniques that can help you unwind and achieve a restful night's sleep.

Regulating the Nervous System

Effective sleep requires more than just a comfortable bed and a dark room; it also involves preparing the mind and body to transition from wakefulness to rest. This preparation is closely tied to the regulation of the nervous system, particularly the ability to exit the "fight or flight" state and enter a state conducive to sleep.

The Fight or Flight Response

The "fight or flight" response is the body's natural reaction to stress, involving the release of stress hormones like cortisol and adrenaline. This response increases heart rate, blood pressure, and energy supplies, preparing the body to deal with perceived threats. While this response is crucial for survival, prolonged activation due to chronic stress can hinder the ability to relax and fall asleep. All of the relaxation strategies in this chapter will help to exit the "fight or flight" response and help to manage stress overall.

Exercise

Exercise is a highly effective strategy for reducing stress and improving sleep quality. Regular physical activity has numerous benefits for both mental and physical health, contributing to a more restful and restorative sleep.

Stress Reduction Through Exercise

Exercise helps reduce stress by lowering levels of the body's stress hormones, such as adrenaline and cortisol. It also stimulates the production of endorphins, chemicals in the brain that act as natural painkillers and mood elevators. Engaging in physical activity can help distract the mind from daily worries, allowing you to unwind and clear your head. Activities such as jogging, swimming, cycling, or even a brisk walk can reduce anxiety and improve mood, making it easier to relax as bedtime approaches.

Improved Sleep Quality

Regular exercise can enhance sleep quality in several ways. First, it helps regulate the circadian rhythm, the body's internal clock that dictates sleep-wake cycles. Exposure to natural light during outdoor exercise further supports this regulation, reinforcing the natural cycle of sleep and wakefulness. Exercise also increases the time spent in deep sleep, the most physically restorative sleep phase. Deep sleep is crucial for the body's recovery processes, including muscle repair and immune function. Moreover, exercise can help alleviate symptoms of sleep disorders such as insomnia and sleep apnea. Studies have shown that people who engage in regular physical activity fall asleep faster, sleep longer, and experience better sleep quality compared to those who do not exercise regularly.

Timing of Exercise

While exercise is beneficial for sleep, the timing of workouts is important. Exercising too close to bedtime can increase adrenaline levels and body temperature, making it harder to fall asleep. Therefore, it's recommended to complete vigorous exercise at least a few hours before bedtime. However, light to moderate activities like yoga or stretching can be done closer to bedtime as they can promote relaxation and help prepare the body for sleep.

Incorporating regular exercise into your routine is a powerful way to reduce stress and improve sleep. By engaging in physical activity, you can enhance both mental and physical health, leading to more restful and restorative sleep.

Meditation and Breathing

Meditation and Breathing Practices for Sleep

Meditation and breathing exercises are powerful tools for promoting relaxation and preparing the mind and body for sleep. These practices help calm the mind, reduce stress, and regulate the nervous system, making it easier to transition into a restful state.

How Meditation Promotes Relaxation

Meditation involves focusing the mind on a particular object, thought, or activity to achieve a mentally clear and emotionally calm state. Regular practice of meditation has been shown to reduce stress, anxiety, and symptoms of depression, all of which can interfere with sleep. By encouraging a state of deep relaxation, meditation helps to quiet the mind, reducing the mental chatter that often keeps people awake at night.

One popular form of meditation for sleep is mindfulness meditation. This practice involves paying attention to the present moment without judgment, often by focusing on the breath or bodily sensations. Studies have demonstrated that mindfulness meditation can improve sleep quality by promoting relaxation and reducing the impact of stress and anxiety on sleep.

Benefits of Breathing Exercises

Breathing exercises are another effective method for promoting relaxation and preparing for sleep. These exercises work by activating the parasympathetic nervous system, which is responsible for the body's rest-and-digest response. Deep, slow breathing can help lower heart rate, reduce blood pressure, and decrease levels of stress hormones, creating a state of calm that is conducive to sleep.

One common breathing technique is diaphragmatic breathing, also known as belly breathing. This involves breathing deeply into the abdomen rather than the chest, which can help maximize oxygen intake and promote relaxation. Another effective method is the 4-7-8 breathing technique, which involves inhaling for four seconds, holding the breath for seven seconds, and exhaling for eight seconds. This pattern helps to slow the breath and induce a state of relaxation.

Combining Meditation and Breathing for Better Sleep

Combining meditation and breathing exercises can enhance their individual benefits and provide a powerful means of preparing for sleep. A simple routine might involve spending a few minutes practicing mindfulness meditation followed by several rounds of deep breathing exercises. This combination can help to clear the mind, reduce physical tension, and signal to the body that it is time to wind down and prepare for sleep.

Practical Tips for Incorporating Meditation and Breathing into Your Routine

Create a Calm Environment: Find a quiet, comfortable space where you won't be disturbed. Dim the lights and remove any distractions.

Set Aside Time: Dedicate 10-20 minutes each evening for meditation and breathing exercises. Consistency is key to reaping the benefits.

Use Guided Resources: If you're new to meditation or breathing exercises, consider using guided meditations or apps designed to help you get started.

Be Patient: It may take some time to feel the full benefits of these practices. Be patient with yourself and keep practicing regularly.

By incorporating meditation and breathing exercises into your nightly routine, you can promote relaxation, reduce stress, and prepare your mind and body for a restful night's sleep.

The Importance of Stress Reduction

Reducing stress is essential for achieving restful sleep, and there are several effective strategies to manage stress throughout the day and before bed. Regular exercise is a powerful way to reduce stress. Physical activity increases the production of endorphins, which are natural mood lifters, and helps decrease levels of anxiety and depression. Activities such as walking, jogging, yoga, and swimming can improve sleep quality by reducing stress levels. Aim for at least 30 minutes of moderate exercise most days of the week.

Maintaining a balanced diet also impacts stress levels and overall health. Consuming a variety of fruits, vegetables, lean proteins, and whole grains provides the necessary nutrients to keep the body functioning optimally. It's important to avoid excessive caffeine and sugar, which can contribute to anxiety and sleep disturbances. Staying hydrated by drinking enough water throughout the day can also help manage stress and support overall health.

Practicing time management by organizing your day and prioritizing tasks can significantly reduce feelings of being overwhelmed. Breaking down large tasks into smaller, manageable steps and setting realistic deadlines can enhance productivity and reduce stress.

Mindfulness and relaxation techniques such as mindfulness meditation, progressive muscle relaxation, and guided imagery can help calm the mind and reduce physical tension. These practices lower cortisol levels and promote relaxation, making it easier to fall asleep.

Journaling before bed can also help clear the mind and reduce anxiety by providing an outlet for expressing emotions and processing the day's events. Additionally, writing down your thoughts or to-do list before bed can help offload worries and prevent them from interfering with sleep .

Clearing the mind of racing thoughts is essential for preparing for sleep. Engaging in calming activities before bed, such as reading a book, listening to soothing music, or practicing gentle yoga, can help clear the mind. Creating a pre-sleep routine that includes these activities can signal to your brain that it's time to wind down.

9

Getting Ready to Sleep

Creating an effective bedtime strategy can significantly improve sleep quality. This chapter outlines a bedtime routine that has worked for me, which can be adapted to suit individual needs. This strategy involves specific steps taken at different times before bed to ensure a restful night's sleep.

3 Hours Before Bed

Eat Final Meal

Having your last meal three hours before bedtime can help avoid indigestion and promote better sleep. Eating too close to bedtime can lead to discomfort and digestive issues, which can interfere with the ability to fall asleep. Opt for a balanced meal with moderate portions to ensure you are not too hungry or too full when you go to bed.

Taper Off Water

Reducing fluid intake in the evening helps minimize nighttime trips to the bathroom. Begin tapering off water consumption three hours before bed to allow your body to process and excrete the excess fluids before you sleep. This practice can help prevent sleep disruptions caused by the need to urinate during the night.

1-2 Hours Before Bed

Take a Hot Bath or Shower

Taking a hot bath or shower an hour or two before bed can promote relaxation and prepare your body for sleep. The rise in body temperature followed by a rapid cooldown mimics the natural temperature drop that occurs before sleep, signaling to your body that it is time to rest.

Drink a Hot Beverage

Consuming a warm, non-caffeinated beverage like herbal tea or bone broth can be soothing and help you unwind. These beverages can provide comfort and help signal to your body that it is time to start winding down. Avoid caffeinated drinks, as they can interfere with sleep.

Limit Blue Light Exposure

Reducing exposure to blue light from screens can help promote melatonin production and prepare your body for sleep. Turn off the TV and set your phone to "Do Not Disturb" mode at least an hour before bed. Consider using blue light blocking glasses if you need to use electronic devices in the evening.

At Bedtime

Meditation and Breathing Exercises

Engage in meditation or deep breathing exercises to calm your mind and relax your body. Techniques such as mindfulness meditation, progressive muscle relaxation, or the 4-7-8 breathing method can help reduce stress and promote a state of relaxation conducive to sleep.

Sleep in a Cool, Completely Dark Room

Ensure your sleeping environment is cool and completely dark. A cool room temperature supports the body's natural thermoregulation process, and complete darkness promotes melatonin production. Use blackout curtains, eye masks, or white noise machines to eliminate light and noise disturbances.

Additional Strategies

Binaural Beats

Listening to binaural beats can help induce relaxation and improve sleep quality. These auditory illusions are created by playing slightly different frequencies in each ear, which can promote brainwave states associated with relaxation and sleep.

Bedtime Stories

Listening to calming bedtime stories can help distract your mind from stressors and create a relaxing bedtime ritual. Audiobooks or guided sleep stories designed for adults can be particularly effective.

White/Gray/Brown Noise

Using white, gray, or brown noise machines can help mask background sounds and create a consistent auditory environment that promotes sleep. These noise types provide different frequency ranges, so you can choose the one that works best for you.

Wake Up with the Sun (or at Sunrise)

Programmed Lights

Using programmable lights that mimic the sunrise can help you wake up naturally and feel more refreshed. These lights gradually increase in brightness, signaling to your body that it is time to wake up. It's best to keep a consistent sleep-wake cycle and using programmed lighting options can help as sunrise varies throughout the year.

Don't Linger in Bed

Getting out of bed promptly after waking can help reinforce a consistent sleep-wake schedule. Avoid staying in bed to snooze, as this can disrupt your sleep pattern and make it harder to wake up feeling refreshed.

Watch the Sunrise

Spending time outside in natural light in the morning helps regulate your circadian rhythm and improve overall sleep quality. Watching the sunrise or exposing yourself to morning light can help reset your internal clock and promote better sleep at night.

By following this bedtime strategy, you can create a routine that promotes relaxation and improves sleep quality. Adapt these steps to suit your individual needs and preferences, and enjoy the benefits of a restful night's sleep.

A Note for Shift Workers

There is no substitute for the natural rising and setting of the sun and this book is targeted to regain that more natural state. However, most of the strategies are effective at enhancing sleep quality no matter when you sleep. If you work third shift, consider using timed and colored lighting to mimic sunrise and sunset whenever you start and end your day.

10

Conclusion

In this book, we've explored various strategies and insights to help you overcome insomnia and achieve restful sleep. From understanding the impact of artificial light and stimulants to implementing effective relaxation techniques and bedtime routines, each chapter has provided practical advice to improve your sleep quality.

We began by defining insomnia and identifying its symptoms and impacts on daily life. Recognizing the difference between sedation from alcohol and achieving restorative sleep highlighted the importance of natural, uninterrupted sleep cycles. We discussed how our modern lifestyle, filled with artificial light and technology, disrupts our circadian rhythms, and how shift work further exacerbates this misalignment. We also examined the role of diet, hydration, and the detrimental effects of caffeine and energy drinks on sleep.

We discussed resetting your internal clock, and that by incorporating relaxation strategies such as exercise, meditation, and stress reduction techniques, you can create a calming pre-sleep routine that helps regulate your nervous system and prepare your mind and body for rest.

Creating a sleep-friendly environment by limiting blue light exposure, maintaining a cool and dark bedroom, and using white noise or binaural beats can further enhance sleep quality. Lastly, a structured bedtime routine, including mindful activities and consistent sleep-wake times, ensures a smooth transition into restful sleep.

Implementing these strategies requires consistency and patience, but the benefits to your overall health and well-being are immense. Better sleep can lead to improved mood, increased productivity, and a greater sense of vitality and balance in your life.

As you continue on your journey to better sleep, I encourage you to experiment with these techniques and find what works best for you. Everyone's sleep needs and preferences are unique, so tailor these recommendations to fit your lifestyle and circumstances.

If you found this book helpful, please consider leaving a review on Amazon. Your feedback is invaluable and helps others who are struggling with insomnia find the tools and strategies they need to improve their sleep. Thank you for taking the time to read this book, and I wish you many nights of restful, restorative sleep.

11

References

American Sleep Apnea Association. (2023, May 30). Understanding sleep cycles and stages - SleepHealth. SleepHealth. https://www.sleephealth.org/sleep-health/importance-of-sleep-understanding-sleep-stages/

Bryan, L., & Singh, A. (2024, May 7). Alcohol and Sleep. sleepfoundation.org. https://www.sleepfoundation.org/nutrition/alcohol-and-sleep

Exercising for better sleep. (2021, August 8). Johns Hopkins Medicine. https://www.hopkinsmedicine.org/health/wellness-and-prevention/exercising-for-better-sleep

Gardiner, C., Weakley, J., Burke, L. M., Roach, G. D., Sargent, C., Maniar, N., Townshend, A., & Halson, S. L. (2023). The effect of caffeine on subsequent sleep: A systematic review and meta-analysis. Sleep Medicine Reviews, 69, 101764. https://doi.org/10.1016/j.smrv.2023.101764

Su, H., Xiao, L., Ren, Y., Xie, H., & Sun, X. (2021). Effects of mindful breathing combined with sleep-inducing exercises in patients with insomnia. World Journal of Clinical Cases, 9(29), 8740–8748. https://doi.org/10.12998/wjcc.v9.i29.8740

Summer, J., & Summer, J. (2024, May 10). Nutrition and Sleep: Diet's Effect on sleep. Sleep Foundation. https://www.sleepfoundation.org/nutrition

Suni, E., & Suni, E. (2023, November 8). Light and sleep. Sleep Foundation. https://www.sleepfoundation.org/bedroom-environment/light-and-sleep

Vogel, K. (2024, March 6). Study: Even the occasional energy drink can increase the risk of sleep disturbances. Health. https://www.health.com/energy-drinks-insomnia-poor-sleep-8550005#:~:text=Researchers%20found%20that%20the%20more,didn't%20drink%20as%20much.

OpenAI. (2024). ChatGPT (July 2024 version) [Large language model]. Retrieved from https://www.openai.com/chatgpt